Vestibular Migraine

A Practical 5-Step Plan to Managing Dizziness Through Diet and Natural Strategies

mf

Disclaimer

This guide is provided for informational and educational purposes only and should not be interpreted as medical, nutritional, or professional advice. The author is not a licensed physician, nurse, dietitian, or mental health provider. Reading this guide does not establish a patient–provider relationship of any kind.

Always seek the guidance of a qualified healthcare professional before starting, changing, or discontinuing any supplement, diet, or lifestyle program. If you are pregnant, breastfeeding, managing a chronic medical condition, or taking prescription medications, consult your physician or pharmacist before considering any product mentioned in this guide.

The author and publisher make no representations or warranties regarding accuracy, applicability, fitness, or completeness of the information contained herein. While every effort has been made to ensure scientific accuracy and currency, medical knowledge and research evolve continually. Readers are responsible for verifying information and making decisions in consultation with licensed professionals.

Use of this guide and any information contained within it is at your own risk. The author and publisher disclaim all liability for any loss, injury, or adverse outcome that may result from the use or misuse of this material.

No supplement, diet, or practice discussed in this text is intended to diagnose, treat, cure, or prevent any disease. No outcomes or benefits are guaranteed.

Product names, supplement formulations, diet frameworks, and trademarks mentioned are the property of their respective owners and are used for identification only. Any images or illustrations that appear in related materials are licensed stock or educational placeholders.

Table of Contents

Introduction

Vestibular migraine is a complex and often misunderstood neurological condition that can significantly disrupt daily life. Unlike typical migraines, vestibular migraine is primarily characterized by recurring episodes of dizziness, vertigo, balance difficulties, and spatial disorientation. Notably, these symptoms can occur with or without the classic migraine headache, which often makes the condition hard to recognize and diagnose accurately without specialized medical input.

The effects of vestibular migraine go far beyond occasional dizziness. Many individuals experience overwhelming unsteadiness, pronounced nausea, hypersensitivity to light and sound, and cognitive symptoms such as brain fog. These challenges can interfere with simple tasks, sometimes leading to missed workdays, reduced social engagement, and even feelings of isolation. The overlap of vestibular migraine symptoms with those of other vestibular and neurological disorders often results in a prolonged process of misdiagnosis or treatment by trial and error, which can be both discouraging and exhausting. Many patients find that clear answers and effective solutions are not always readily available, as clinical protocols for vestibular migraine continue to develop.

Traditional treatment for vestibular migraine has relied on medications such as anti-vertigo drugs, beta blockers, antidepressants, or anticonvulsants. While some individuals benefit from these medications, others find them ineffective, develop adverse reactions, or notice diminishing results over time. Moreover, long-term medication use can carry unwanted side effects or interact with other health issues. These limitations have prompted increased interest in alternative approaches, including dietary changes, lifestyle modifications, and natural interventions.

Non-pharmaceutical strategies are now recognized as an essential part of managing vestibular migraine. For example, certain foods and additives, such as caffeine, aged cheeses, chocolate, and flavor enhancers like MSG, can trigger symptoms in some people. Skipping meals, dehydration, and a lack of essential nutrients can further increase susceptibility to dizziness and neurological disturbances. Proactive planning around nutrition, hydration, and regular meal timing has become a cornerstone of effective management. Additionally, holistic measures such as vestibular rehabilitation exercises, stress-reduction techniques, and targeted supplementation can help individuals regain control and find sustainable relief.

In this guide, you will find:

- Straightforward explanations of the science behind vestibular migraine, helping you understand what's happening in your body.
- Proven strategies for identifying your personal migraine triggers, empowering you to take control of your health.
- An easy-to-follow five-step dietary plan, specifically designed to support vestibular health.
- Natural techniques for relieving symptoms, so you can find comfort during flare-ups.
- Guidance on building a supportive mindset for long-term change, fostering resilience and positivity.
- Insights into the importance of small yet powerful daily habits that contribute to lasting improvement.
- Trusted resources for ongoing support, ensuring you have reliable information and a sense of community.

Following the recommendations and frameworks presented here, you can gain practical strategies to reduce your symptoms and reclaim your quality of life. Remember that there are various options available to support you throughout this process.

Vestibular Migraine Fundamentals

For many, the journey toward better vestibular migraine management begins with a need for understanding. The frustration and confusion of navigating vague or shifting symptoms can feel isolating. This chapter offers clarity by unpacking the unique science and diagnostic features of vestibular migraine. By grounding yourself in these fundamentals, you will be prepared to make sense of later guidance on triggers, diet, and self-care.

Defining vestibular migraine and its unique neurological mechanisms

Vestibular migraine is a neurological disorder marked by intermittent disturbances in balance and perception of space. While migraine is typically associated with recurring headaches, vestibular migraine often causes dizziness, vertigo (the sensation that you or your environment is spinning), unsteadiness, and visual disturbances, with or without the presence of a classic migraine headache.

What sets vestibular migraine apart from other types of migraine is its direct involvement with the brain's vestibular system. The vestibular system is responsible for processing information about motion, balance, and spatial orientation. In people with vestibular migraine, changes in brain activity can transiently disrupt the normal operation of this system. This may result in profound sensations of movement, imbalance, or even a feeling that the ground is shifting beneath you.

Neurologically, vestibular migraine is thought to arise from a mix of genetic predisposition and altered brain signaling. Migraine pathways involve abnormal activation in the brainstem and altered neurotransmitter levels, especially regarding serotonin and calcitonin gene-related peptide (CGRP). When these migraine-related processes affect the networks that communicate with the inner ear and cerebellum (the balance centers in the brain), vestibular symptoms emerge. Notably, these disruptions may occur with little or no headache, which can complicate both recognition and diagnosis.

Prevalence estimates and population groups most affected

Although vestibular migraine has gained more recognition in recent years, its exact prevalence remains difficult to measure due to challenges with underdiagnosis and inconsistent diagnostic criteria. Recent research indicates that vestibular migraine likely affects around 1% of the general population. However, among individuals already diagnosed with migraine, the prevalence is substantially higher, with estimates suggesting that 9 to 10% of migraine sufferers experience vestibular migraine symptoms at some point in their lives.

Vestibular migraine can develop at any age, but most cases are identified in adults between 30 and 50 years old. The condition is notably more common in women, occurring two to three times more frequently than in men. This gender disparity is thought to be related to hormonal influences, particularly the impact of estrogen fluctuations on both migraine and vestibular symptoms.

Several factors influence who is most affected by vestibular migraine. These include:

1. ***Age***: While vestibular migraine can present at any stage of life, it is most commonly diagnosed in middle-aged adults, particularly those in their thirties and forties.
2. ***Gender***: Women are at significantly greater risk compared to men. Hormonal changes, such as those occurring during menstruation, pregnancy, or menopause, are believed to contribute to this increased susceptibility.

3. ***Family History***: There is a strong genetic component, with many patients reporting a family history of either vestibular migraine or classic migraine.
4. ***Ethnic and Geographic Distribution***: The condition has been observed across various ethnic groups and in both urban and rural populations. However, differences in access to healthcare and specialists can influence the rates at which vestibular migraine is diagnosed.

Understanding which groups are most at risk is essential for improving recognition and diagnosis of vestibular migraine. As awareness grows, it becomes increasingly important to identify the distinguishing features of vestibular migraine, especially in comparison with other disorders that cause dizziness or vertigo.

Core symptoms and differentiating features from other vestibular disorders

The hallmark of vestibular migraine is a recurring pattern of vestibular (balance-related) symptoms that may last from minutes to several days. **Typical experiences include:**

- ***Spontaneous vertigo attacks***: Sudden episodes of spinning or motion, occurring without warning.
- Persistent sense of unsteadiness or ***loss of balance***.
- ***Motion sensitivity***: Feeling worse during or after head movement, changes in posture, walking in busy environments, or traveling in vehicles.

- ***Visual discomfort***: Difficulty tolerating bright lights (photophobia), visual patterns, or complex environments like crowded supermarkets.
- ***Nausea and sometimes vomiting***, often accompanying the vertigo or dizziness.
- ***Changes in hearing or ear symptoms***, such as feeling of fullness in the ears or mild tinnitus.
- ***Cognitive symptoms***: Many people report brain fog, difficulty with concentration, or slowed thinking during an episode.

Unlike other common vestibular conditions (such as benign paroxysmal positional vertigo [BPPV], Ménière's disease, or vestibular neuritis), vestibular migraine typically lacks structural damage to the inner ear. In BPPV, vertigo is almost exclusively triggered by head position changes, while Ménière's disease presents with hearing loss and ringing in the ears as core symptoms. Vestibular migraine, in contrast, is often "multimodal" and episodic, showing up unpredictably and with varying intensity.

One of the main clues suggesting vestibular migraine is the presence of migraine features, such as headache, visual aura, photophobia, or phonophobia, either during or in between dizzy episodes. However, some people never develop head pain at all, while others alternate between classic migraines and vestibular symptoms.

Common challenges in diagnosis and misdiagnosis

Diagnosing vestibular migraine is often far from straightforward. Unlike disorders that show up on a simple blood test or brain scan, vestibular migraine requires careful clinical evaluation and a detailed medical history. **<u>This complexity comes from several factors:</u>**

- ***Symptom overlap***: Many other conditions, from inner ear infections to anxiety disorders, can cause dizziness or vertigo. This overlap makes it easy for vestibular migraine to be mistaken for other vestibular problems, especially if no headache is present.
- ***Fluctuating presentation***: Symptoms can change over time, sometimes appearing mild and at other times intense, making it difficult to capture a clear pattern necessary for diagnosis.
- ***Inconsistent terminology***: Physicians sometimes use different labels, such as "migraine-associated vertigo" or "migrainous vertigo," which can cause confusion for both patients and practitioners.
- ***Variable medical awareness***: Not all healthcare providers are equally familiar with vestibular migraine. Some may focus on the absence of headache, inadvertently ruling out migraine as a possible cause for vestibular symptoms.

Misdiagnosis is common. People are frequently told they have BPPV, Ménière's disease, anxiety, or even psychiatric disorders before the connection to migraine is considered. This can lead to years of ineffective treatments and ongoing distress.

Vestibular Migraine: Core Diagnostic Criteria (adapted from International Headache Society):

1. At least five episodes with vestibular (dizzy/vertigo) symptoms of moderate or severe intensity, lasting 5 minutes to 72 hours.
2. Current or previous history of migraine with or without aura.
3. One or more migraine features during at least half of episodes:
    - Headache with typical migraine characteristics (moderate/severe, one-sided, throbbing, aggravated by movement)
    - Sensitivity to light (photophobia) and/or sound (phonophobia)
    - Visual aura
4. No better explanation for the symptoms.

If you or your healthcare provider use these criteria as a framework during consultations, it may increase the chance of early recognition and more appropriate management. Building from the diagnostic hurdles, it is helpful to understand why vestibular and migraine pathways are so strongly connected in the first place.

The connection between migraine pathways and the vestibular system

Migraines are now recognized as complex neural events involving electrical and chemical changes in the brain. Once triggered, these changes impact parts of the brain responsible for pain, sensory processing, and autonomic function. In vestibular migraine, the disruption specifically reaches brain networks involved in equilibrium, coordination, and spatial orientation.

Neuroscientists believe that abnormal activation of the trigeminal nerve, a major sensory pathway implicated in all migraine types, may influence both blood vessel tone and neurotransmitter release in neighboring areas that control balance. Fluctuations in serotonin and CGRP (a protein that triggers inflammation and transmission of pain signals) modulate not only headache pain but also affect the vestibular nuclei, which are clusters of nerve cells coordinating signals from the inner ear to the brain.

This explains why vestibular symptoms can occur independently or alongside head pain. In some cases, the migraine "storm" primarily disturbs the balance centers, leading to vertigo or unsteadiness, while in others, it follows a more traditional pain-dominated pattern.

Triggers such as hormonal changes, stress, dehydration, skipped meals, or exposure to certain foods can set off these cascades. When the brain is hypersensitive due to chronic migraine activity, even minor provocations, such as a bright light or sudden movement, may tip the balance into a full-blown episode.

Viewing vestibular migraine not just as a variant of headache disorder, but as a whole-brain sensitivity problem with unique effects on the body's sense of position and motion, opens a clearer path to personalized management.

As you move forward, an accurate understanding of your own symptoms and potential triggers is critical. Later chapters will guide you in capturing this information and using it to shape your plan. For now, building this foundational knowledge positions you to communicate more effectively with healthcare providers and make informed choices about your care.

Identifying and Tracking Your Personal Triggers

Understanding the patterns behind your vestibular migraine symptoms can feel like solving a complex puzzle. Yet, knowing what sets off your dizziness, vertigo, or discomfort is one of the most powerful things you can do for self-management. The process begins with identifying your personal triggers, those factors in your daily life that set the stage for an episode. This chapter will guide you through broad category triggers, practical methods for meticulous tracking, and how to recognize patterns that lead to meaningful changes.

Broad Categories of Vestibular Migraine Triggers

Triggers for vestibular migraine are highly individual, but most fall into a few main categories: dietary, environmental, hormonal, and sleep-related. Recognizing these categories is a helpful starting point as you begin to decipher what prompts your symptoms.

1. ***Dietary triggers are among the most researched.*** Certain foods and food additives have a reputation for provoking migraine episodes in sensitive individuals. These include aged cheeses, processed meats containing nitrates, chocolate, foods with monosodium glutamate (MSG), alcohol (especially red wine), and artificial sweeteners like aspartame. Beverages with caffeine, especially when consumed inconsistently, can both trigger and relieve migraine attacks, which can cause confusion about their real impact. Skipping meals or inconsistent eating patterns can also destabilize your system, particularly if blood sugar drops.
2. ***Environmental triggers span a wide range***, from changes in weather or barometric pressure to exposure to strong odors, flickering or fluorescent lights, loud noises, and visual "busy-ness" like crowded places. Rapid shifts in altitude, humidity, or temperature may also exacerbate symptoms. Even subtle stressors, such as a long car ride or scrolling quickly through digital screens, can challenge your vestibular system and provoke symptoms for some people.
3. ***Hormonal triggers are especially relevant for women.*** Many report worsening of symptoms during menstruation, ovulation, or menopause. Fluctuations in estrogen are thought to influence not only headache-type migraines but vestibular events as well.

For some, hormone replacement therapy or certain birth control methods can either aggravate or stabilize symptoms. Men are not immune, as any significant change in the body's internal chemistry, whether due to thyroid fluctuations, illness, or stress, can play a part.

4. ***Sleep-related triggers are crucial but often overlooked.*** Both lack of sleep and oversleeping may disrupt the delicate equilibrium in the brain's migraine pathways. Poor-quality sleep, frequent nighttime awakenings, or working irregular shifts may leave you much more vulnerable to dizziness and vertigo. Recognizing the cumulative impact of "sleep debt" or inconsistency is key to managing vestibular symptoms long-term.

Understanding these broad categories of vestibular migraine triggers can empower you to identify patterns in your own symptoms. Through careful observation and lifestyle adjustments, you may reduce the frequency and severity of your episodes.

Keeping a detailed symptom and food diary

The first actionable step in identifying your triggers is to document your experiences consistently and carefully. A combined symptom and food diary serves as the cornerstone of self-discovery.

To get started, choose a format you will actually use: a paper notebook, a printed template, or a digital document. **Each day, note the following:**

- Every meal, beverage, and snack you consume, including the specific time.
- Any episodes of dizziness, vertigo, imbalance, nausea, visual disturbances, or new neurological symptoms.
- The severity of each symptom (1-10 scale is common).
- Non-dietary factors present (e.g., weather changes, stress levels, locations visited, menstrual cycle phase, sleep quality).
- Any new medications or supplements taken.

Try to make notes in real-time or as closely as possible; details can fade quickly, especially when you're not feeling well. Reviewing even one or two weeks of daily records can be eye-opening. Patterns may begin to emerge, such as headaches after certain foods or increased dizziness following disrupted sleep.

To make your diary more effective:

- Be honest and thorough, even when a meal or moment feels insignificant. Triggers are sometimes subtle or cumulative.
- Include context like travel, social events, or unusual days because these often coincide with symptom flares.

- Use abbreviations or checkboxes if that saves you time, but don't skip on details where possible.

This log will act as a personal data set, offering clues and trends specific to you rather than relying solely on general lists of "common" triggers.

Recognizing Dietary, Environmental, Hormonal, and Sleep Triggers

Once your diary has at least two to four weeks of entries, review the records for recurring patterns:

- Are symptoms more common after certain foods or beverages? For example, do dizzy spells follow days when you had wine, MSG, or missed breakfast?
- Do attacks cluster during your menstrual cycle, before periods, or during ovulation?
- Are there environmental or sensory exposures that link to your symptoms, such as after long drives, exposure to fluorescent lights, or after a day with dramatic weather changes?
- Does sleep disruption (late nights, sleeping in, or restless nights) precede symptom flares?

Sometimes, triggers work in combination. Perhaps you're fine with a glass of wine on a restful weekend, but if you also had a poor night's sleep and ate a high-sodium meal, an episode follows. Tracking all aspects, including dietary, environmental, hormonal, and sleep, lets you see these nuances.

When patterns are unclear, try a short-term "elimination test": remove one suspected trigger at a time for several weeks, note your symptoms, then reintroduce it to see if attacks reoccur. This can be very telling for foods, beverages, or lifestyle habits.

For women, tracking your symptoms alongside your menstrual cycle can offer especially valuable insights. Some use color-coding or symbols to coordinate symptom records with cycle phases, making it easier to spot hormonal influences. Similarly, log minor illnesses, medication changes, or major life events because they may play a role you hadn't considered.

Using tracking apps and checklists for pattern recognition

While pen-and-paper tracking works for many, a range of digital tools and apps can make the process easier and more powerful. Apps often include built-in reminders, customizable trackers, and data visualization to help you spot trends you might otherwise miss.

Some popular app features for migraine and vestibular symptom tracking:

- Daily logs for food, water intake, sleep, physical activity, and menstrual cycles.
- Symptom scoring and timing, with options to add environmental factors or stress ratings.
- Automated graphs and reports showing symptom frequency, severity, and potential associations.
- Medication, supplement, and menstrual trackers integrated for completeness.

Apps like Migraine Buddy, Headache Diary Pro, or general health tracking tools allow you to export your data for review, share it with healthcare providers, and often receive notifications if certain thresholds are crossed.

Checklists are another practical strategy. You can create a physical or digital list of common triggers, such as foods, setting factors, stressors, and more. At the end of each day, check off which ones you encountered. Soon, it becomes easier to see at a glance what triggers were present, even on busy or overwhelming days. The key is consistency: whichever system you choose, stick to it for at least a full month. Data becomes more reliable as you continue, and the cumulative picture is far richer than any single day's experience.

Interpreting Trigger Data for Actionable Insights

All of your careful tracking and record-keeping comes together in an important phase: using your data to make meaningful changes. Recognizing patterns allows you to find insights that can help prevent or reduce vestibular migraine episodes, moving beyond just documentation.

Begin by searching for the most frequent correlations in your data. For example, you might observe:

- Dizziness occurs after eating processed meats on three out of four occasions.
- Vertigo is most intense two days before menstruation.
- Attacks tend to cluster after three consecutive nights of poor sleep.
- Weekends, with less structure and irregular meal times, consistently lead to increased symptoms.

Take your time with this process. It may require several cycles or seasons to notice trends related to weather or hormones. Exporting your tracking data into simple spreadsheets or creating graphs of symptom frequency can help you visualize subtle connections that might otherwise go unnoticed.

Once likely culprits are identified, the next step is practical experimentation:

- Remove or reduce a suspected trigger for a minimum of two weeks (for foods, aim for three to four weeks).
- Maintain all other routines and diary methods.
- If symptoms decrease, cautiously reintroduce the item and monitor your response.
- If symptoms spike again, that trigger is likely significant, and sustained avoidance may be wise.

Keep in mind, triggers are addictive. Managing as many as possible, even those with minor effects, often delivers the greatest benefit. Sometimes, your tracking reveals that certain factors (such as fluctuating light patterns or cyclical hormonal changes) cannot be fully controlled. For these, plan around them: maintain extra hydration, consistent meals, and reduce exposure to other triggers during vulnerable times.

Share your insights with healthcare providers, family members, or support groups. Your personalized trigger profile is a roadmap, not just for management but for empowering discussions about your needs and accommodations as you progress through your action plan. Approaching your vestibular migraine triggers methodically through recording, reviewing, experimenting, and acting, you lay the foundation for the natural management strategies outlined in the next chapters. One step at a time, you will transform daunting uncertainty into informed and proactive self-care.

Core Principles of the Vestibular Migraine Diet

For many living with vestibular migraine, dietary strategy is a crucial pillar of symptom control. The right approach can reduce dizziness, improve stability, and restore a better quality of life. Before adopting specific meal plans, it's helpful to understand the core principles underlying a vestibular migraine-friendly diet. This chapter covers the scientific rationale for dietary changes, tips for recognizing and eliminating triggers, the importance of consistent habits, key micronutrients, and how to assemble balanced, anti-inflammatory meals for lasting support.

Migraine-friendly diet overview and its scientific rationale

A migraine-friendly diet is based on the understanding that specific foods and additives can impact the brain's excitability and provoke migraine attacks, including those that involve the vestibular system. Research indicates that dietary triggers contribute to migraine pathophysiology through mechanisms like blood vessel dilation, changes in neurotransmitters (particularly serotonin), and activation of inflammatory pathways. People with migraine tend to have brains that are especially responsive to these external chemical and nutritional signals.

Well-known dietary triggers include aged cheeses, processed meats, monosodium glutamate (MSG), chocolate, alcohol (especially red wine), and foods containing artificial sweeteners or preservatives. Caffeine, as well as foods rich in tyramine or nitrates, are frequently cited as potential triggers. These substances may induce cortical spreading depression (a key event in migraine), influence vascular tone, or disturb normal neurotransmitter activity.

On the other hand, a purposeful, nutrient-dense diet can help protect against migraine attacks. Maintaining regular meal times, staying hydrated, and steering clear of personal dietary triggers support greater stability in the brain and nervous system, reducing the likelihood of vestibular disturbances. Through thoughtful nutritional choices, it is possible to ease neurological hypersensitivity and encourage more consistent brain function.

Identifying and eliminating dietary triggers

Awareness of personal food triggers is central to the vestibular migraine diet. While research-backed lists of common triggers provide a starting point, not every person reacts to the same foods because individual variability is the rule. As emphasized in the previous chapter, tracking your symptoms alongside food intake is the best way to determine which items, if any, exacerbate your dizziness, vertigo, or other migraine symptoms. The standard first step is to eliminate known common triggers from your diet for a period of at least 2–4 weeks. **Top offenders often include:**

- Aged cheeses (such as cheddar, blue cheese, parmesan)
- Processed meats (salami, hot dogs, ham)
- Chocolate
- Nuts and nut butters
- Red wine and dark spirits
- Beer (especially those containing yeast)
- Foods with MSG (such as some Asian cuisines, snack foods, and seasonings)
- Fermented foods (sauerkraut, pickles, certain yogurts)
- Artificial sweeteners (aspartame, sucralose)
- Caffeinated beverages in excess

The elimination phase can feel daunting, but it allows you to pinpoint sensitivities by then gradually reintroducing items one at a time and monitoring your body's responses. During this process, pay attention to:

- The timing of symptoms relative to food consumption (typically within 24 hours)
- Delayed or cumulative effects (some triggers may take several exposures)

- Combined triggers (two mildly problematic foods may provoke more symptoms together than alone)

Document your findings so you and your healthcare team can make informed choices about permanent dietary adjustments.

Structuring consistent meal timing and hydration routines

Inconsistency in meal patterning can itself be a significant trigger for vestibular migraine. Skipping meals, long fasting intervals, or erratic eating disrupt blood sugar stability, which is associated with increased cortical and vestibular sensitivity. For people with migraine, these rapid changes in metabolism can easily tip the nervous system into an episode.

To establish a migraine-friendly routine, aim for:

- Eating balanced meals and small snacks at regular intervals (every 3–4 hours during waking hours)
- Avoiding skipped meals, even on busy days or when not feeling hungry
- Pairing carbohydrates with protein or healthy fats to slow absorption and maintain blood sugar stability

Hydration is equally important, as dehydration is a well-known migraine trigger and can worsen symptoms like dizziness and lightheadedness. **General hydration guidelines include:**

- Drinking water steadily throughout the day (not just in large amounts at once)
- Avoiding or limiting beverages that act as diuretics, such as caffeinated energy drinks or large quantities of black tea and coffee
- Including electrolyte-rich fluids in your diet, particularly if you are physically active or lose fluids through sweating (good sources include coconut water, naturally flavored water, or balanced electrolyte solutions without excessive sugar)

Developing routines, such as setting reminders, carrying a water bottle, and packing portable snacks, helps ensure these supportive habits become effortless over time.

Essential micronutrients for vestibular and neurological health

Deficiencies in several vitamins and minerals have been linked with increased migraine frequency and severity, including vestibular subtypes. Correcting these deficiencies can therefore be an important part of a comprehensive dietary plan.

1. **Magnesium**

   is one of the best-studied micronutrients in migraine prevention. It plays a role in nerve signal transmission, neurovascular stability, and moderating excitotoxicity;

all of which matter in controlling vestibular symptoms. Low magnesium levels are associated with increased migraine attack frequency, and supplementation, typically around 400 mg per day and adjusted individually, is often recommended for migraine sufferers.

2. **Riboflavin (vitamin B2)**

   is involved in mitochondrial energy metabolism. Insufficient riboflavin can decrease cellular energy, potentially increasing migraine vulnerability. Studies suggest that daily riboflavin supplementation may help reduce frequency and intensity of migraine attacks, including those of the vestibular type.

3. **Coenzyme Q10 (CoQ10)**

   another mitochondrial cofactor, is gaining research support for its role in preventing migraine by enhancing cellular energy production and defending against oxidative stress. A usual supplemental dose is 100–300 mg daily, though dietary sources (like fatty fish and whole grains) contribute as well.

4. **Vitamin D and omega-3 fatty acids**

   (from sources like salmon, sardines, flaxseed) also play roles in neural protection and immune modulation. Deficiencies in these nutrients correlate with higher rates of migraine and vestibular symptoms.

Key sources of migraine-preventive micronutrients include:

- ***Leafy greens and vegetables***: These provide essential magnesium and B vitamins.
- ***Seeds and nuts***: These are rich in magnesium and healthy fats, though they are only recommended for those not sensitive to them.
- ***Dairy and eggs***: These are excellent sources of riboflavin and vitamin D.
- ***Whole grains***: These contain B vitamins and magnesium.
- ***Fatty fish***: These provide CoQ10 and omega-3s.
- ***Legumes***: These offer magnesium and plant protein.
- ***Fortified foods or supplements***: These are useful for vitamin D intake, especially during winter or times with limited sun exposure.

It's important to work with a healthcare professional to evaluate your nutritional status and discuss safe supplementation where appropriate.

Building a Balanced, Anti-Inflammatory Meal Plan

Developing a meal plan that supports vestibular health involves assembling meals that are nutritionally balanced, anti-inflammatory, and mindful of individual triggers. Rather than focusing on restriction, the goal is to choose foods that nourish the nervous system and help reduce inflammation.

A key aspect of anti-inflammatory eating is emphasizing whole, minimally processed foods. Colorful fruits and vegetables are rich in antioxidants and polyphenols, which help protect nerve tissues from oxidative and inflammatory stress. Lean protein sources, including poultry, fish, legumes, and eggs, supply essential amino acids that support neurotransmitter balance. Healthy fats from olive oil, avocado, and certain seeds contribute to cognitive function and hormonal health.

Sample guidelines for building vestibular migraine-friendly meals:

- Make half your plate vegetables and fruits of various colors, focusing on those high in vitamin C and phytonutrients, such as spinach, bell peppers, berries, and carrots.
- Choose whole grains like brown rice, quinoa, and oats instead of refined carbohydrates.

- Include lean protein according to your personal tolerances, such as chicken, turkey, fish, legumes, or eggs.
- Emphasize healthy fats, including olive oil, avocado, and chia or flaxseed, unless seeds are a trigger.
- Limit added sugars, deep-fried foods, high-sodium packaged items, and processed meats.
- Use herbs and spices instead of salt-heavy or MSG-laden seasonings.

Personalization is key; adjust these recommendations according to your own food triggers and preferences. For example, some people may find that garlic, onions, or certain fruits and vegetables provoke symptoms, while others tolerate them well. A food and symptom diary can be a helpful tool for refining your approach and optimizing results.

A sample day might include:

- ***Breakfast***: Oatmeal with fresh berries and pumpkin seeds, if tolerated, plus a glass of water.
- ***Lunch***: Grilled chicken salad with mixed greens, bell peppers, quinoa, olive oil, and lemon dressing.
- ***Snack***: Sliced apple with sunflower seed butter or coconut yogurt.
- ***Dinner***: Baked salmon, roasted sweet potatoes, and steamed broccoli.
- ***Beverages***: Water, herbal teas, or unsweetened coconut water.

This model is flexible; rotate foods, adjust for individual tolerances, and aim for variety to ensure nutritional adequacy and enjoyment.

Adopting a vestibular migraine diet involves understanding your personal triggers, maintaining consistent routines, and focusing on nutrient-rich, anti-inflammatory foods. These core principles can help reduce symptoms and support overall neurological health. With patience and careful tracking, you can find a sustainable approach that enhances your quality of life.

Step 1 - Foundation: Trigger Elimination and Substitution

Starting a migraine-friendly diet can seem daunting, but understanding the foundational steps will set you up for long-term success. In this step, you'll focus on systematically removing or substituting foods and ingredients that may be linked to vestibular migraine symptoms, while learning to navigate grocery aisles and restaurant menus with confidence. Managing caffeine intake and withdrawal is also important at this stage, as is setting practical expectations to help you stay motivated and on track. Let's break the process down into manageable actions for beginners seeking tangible relief from vestibular migraine.

Systematic Approach to Elimination and Substitution

While Chapter 3 addressed the most common dietary triggers for vestibular symptoms, this chapter is dedicated to helping you put that information into action by developing a personalized and sustainable elimination plan. Rather than making sweeping dietary changes all at once, it is generally more effective to take a stepwise approach. This method can help prevent feelings of overwhelm and allows for the maintenance of proper nutritional balance throughout the process.

A systematic elimination plan typically includes several key steps:

1. Begin by reviewing your food and symptom diary to pinpoint which triggers highlighted in Chapter 3 may be particularly relevant for you. Careful observation can help you identify patterns between specific foods and symptom flare-ups.
2. Next, gradually remove or substitute one or two of the suspected trigger foods at a time. Allow yourself a period of two to four weeks for each change before making additional adjustments. This incremental approach gives your body time to adjust and makes it easier to assess whether symptoms improve.
3. Throughout this process, maintain a detailed symptom log. By recording any changes in the frequency or intensity of dizziness, vertigo, or "cloudy-headed" episodes, you can more accurately track the effects of dietary modifications.
4. If appropriate, consider reintroducing foods one at a time, spacing each new reintroduction several days apart. This careful reintroduction allows you to

determine with greater confidence which foods truly contribute to your symptoms.

Consulting with a registered dietitian or healthcare provider can offer individualized guidance and help you avoid nutritional deficiencies. Many people report a substantial reduction in vestibular symptoms as they fine-tune their diet through this methodical process.

Safe Food Substitution Options for Flavor and Nutrition

Removing familiar foods does not mean sacrificing taste or balanced nutrition. The key is discovering migraine-friendly alternatives that support neurological health without provoking symptoms.

Consider these common substitutions for frequently problematic foods:

- ***Caffeinated coffee***: Decaf, if tolerated, or naturally caffeine-free herbal teas such as chamomile, ginger, or peppermint.
- ***Aged cheeses***: Fresh cheeses like mozzarella, ricotta, cream cheese, or cottage cheese.
- ***Cured meats***: Plain roasted turkey, chicken breast, or freshly prepared lean cuts without added nitrates or preservatives.

- ***MSG and artificial additives***: Natural herbs such as rosemary, thyme, and parsley, or spices, lemon zest, and garlic.
- ***Chocolate***: Baked goods flavored with pure vanilla or carob powder.
- ***Alcohol***: Sparkling water with a splash of natural fruit juice for festive occasions.
- ***Fermented and pickled items***: Fresh vegetables like cucumber, red bell pepper, or tomatoes drizzled with olive oil.

A migraine-friendly plate should include complex carbohydrates, lean proteins, and healthy fats to stabilize blood sugar and support brain function. Quinoa, sweet potato, brown rice, lentils, leafy greens, olive oil, and avocado are nutritious staples to consider.

Experiment with one substitution per week to gradually build a repertoire of satisfying, vestibular-friendly meals.

Navigating Packaged Foods and Restaurant Menus

Packaged foods and restaurant meals often contain hidden triggers, even in options that seem healthy at first glance. Developing the skills to read food labels and communicate your dietary needs effectively when eating out is essential to prevent accidental exposures and maintain your well-being.

When shopping for packaged foods, consider the following steps:

1. **Carefully read ingredient lists on all products.**

   Look for and avoid terms such as "hydrolyzed protein," "yeast extract," "natural flavors," "sodium nitrite/nitrate," or "monosodium glutamate," as these can be common triggers.

2. **Limit your intake of processed snacks**

   Like canned soups, instant noodle meals, condiments, and flavored chips, since these often contain additives or hidden ingredients that may be problematic.

3. **Select items with short, simple ingredient lists.**

   Whenever possible, opt for "plain" or unseasoned versions of foods, which are less likely to contain hidden triggers.

When dining out at restaurants, follow these guidelines:

1. Review menus online ahead of time to identify dishes prepared with simple, whole ingredients.
2. Ask your server how dishes are made, and specifically inquire whether any sauces, dressings, or marinades contain potential triggers.

3. Request modifications to your meal, such as grilled meats without marinade or salads dressed with olive oil and lemon juice instead of pre-made dressings.
4. If you are uncertain about a particular dish, choose the safest option available and communicate your dietary needs clearly to your server. Most restaurants are accustomed to accommodating special dietary requests.

With regular practice, reading labels and navigating menus will become easier, helping you avoid dietary slip-ups and better manage your symptoms.

Managing Caffeine Intake and Withdrawal Symptoms

Caffeine is a well-known migraine trigger, especially when consumption is inconsistent. For many individuals with vestibular migraine, reducing or eliminating caffeine brings notable relief.

If you consume caffeine daily, a gradual reduction helps minimize withdrawal symptoms such as headache, fatigue, irritability, and temporary increases in dizziness. To taper caffeine:

- Reduce daily intake by 25% to 50% every 3 to 5 days, substituting with water, herbal teas, or decaf options.

- Stay hydrated to prevent dehydration-related symptoms.
- Get plenty of rest during the taper period.
- Use gentle remedies, such as a cool compress, for mild headaches.
- If approved by your provider, a low-dose pain reliever, such as acetaminophen, may help during withdrawal.

Caffeine withdrawal rarely lasts more than one to two weeks. Many people report steadier energy and more predictable symptom patterns afterward.

Setting Realistic Expectations for Dietary Changes

Natural management of vestibular migraine through dietary modifications is a gradual process. Setting realistic expectations can prevent frustration and help keep motivation high.

Keep in mind:

- Improvement is often gradual, with reductions in symptom frequency and severity emerging over weeks to months.
- Some fluctuations are normal, especially during periods of stress or poor sleep.
- Not all suspected triggers will be problematic for everyone; personal experimentation is key.
- Social situations may require extra planning, and brief setbacks are learning opportunities, not failures.

Celebrate small wins, such as fewer dizzy episodes or improved concentration. Stay in touch with your healthcare team and track your progress to observe positive trends over time.

In this foundational step, your main goals are to identify which foods and additives may be linked to symptoms, find enjoyable alternatives, and foster habits that support ongoing success in vestibular migraine management. With mindful elimination and thoughtful substitution, you're laying the groundwork for lasting relief and improved quality of life.

Step 2 - Hydration, Electrolyte Balance, and Meal Timing

Feeling dizzy is an all-too-common experience for those dealing with vestibular migraine. Sometimes, the source of that spinning sensation is surprisingly simple: dehydration or erratic eating habits. Many people overlook the powerful role that fluid balance, electrolytes, and steady meal timing play in keeping dizziness and broader migraine symptoms at bay. This chapter offers concrete steps to create a daily routine that minimizes these hidden triggers and supports lasting vestibular stability.

Understanding dehydration's link to dizziness

Dizziness is a hallmark of vestibular migraine, but it is also a classic symptom of dehydration. The body relies on a carefully maintained balance of water and electrolytes to ensure optimal blood flow, nerve conduction, and inner ear function. When hydration levels drop, blood volume decreases with it, leading to lower blood pressure and reduced perfusion of the brain's delicate vestibular system. For someone with vestibular migraine, this may directly increase susceptibility to vertigo, light-headedness, and even increase the risk of a full-blown migraine attack.

Scientific research points out that even mild dehydration can alter how well the vestibular system works, causing or intensifying dizziness sensations. Symptoms such as cotton-mouth, dry skin, concentrated urine, or a slight increase in heart rate can signal that you are already mildly dehydrated and at greater risk for vestibular symptoms. Pay close attention to these subtle signs, as people with migraine may have a heightened sensitivity to any disruption in fluid and mineral balance.

Creating a Hydration Schedule with Optimal Electrolyte Sources

To prevent dehydration from undermining your vestibular health, it helps to build a simple hydration routine into your day. Most adults need between 2 and 3 liters, about 8 to 12 cups, of water and other fluids each day, but individual needs can vary depending on body size, climate, activity level, and specific symptoms. For those with vestibular migraine, consistent hydration throughout the day is crucial; rapidly drinking large amounts of water at once is less effective and can increase the urge to urinate quickly, potentially leading to a net fluid loss.

A hydration schedule is straightforward and can be easily tailored:

- ***On waking***: Drink 1 glass of water, around 250 ml, immediately.
- ***With each meal***: Have 1 to 2 glasses of water, sipping steadily.
- ***Between meals***: Schedule small water breaks every 1 to 2 hours.
- ***Before, during, and after exercise or periods of heat***: Increase fluid intake appropriately.

Good hydration, however, is about more than just water. Electrolytes, which are minerals like sodium, potassium, magnesium, and calcium, help regulate fluid movement between cells, nerve signal transmission, and muscle contraction. Sudden losses of electrolytes from sweating, diarrhea, or certain medications can trigger dizziness, muscle cramps, mental fog, and worsen migraine.

Instead of relying solely on electrolyte drinks marketed for athletes, focus on natural, migraine-safe sources:

- Add a pinch of unrefined sea salt or a few slices of cucumber and lemon to your water for gentle electrolyte enhancement.
- Incorporate potassium-rich foods, such as bananas, oranges, potatoes, and spinach, and magnesium

sources, like pumpkin seeds, almonds, and beans, into your meals.

- If recommended by your healthcare provider, consider using oral rehydration solutions, especially during illness or heat waves.

Avoid sports drinks with artificial colors, added sugars, and preservatives, as these can act as migraine triggers. Homemade infusions or coconut water, in moderation, are often better tolerated.

Role of meal timing in blood sugar regulation

For people living with vestibular migraine, large swings in blood sugar are known instigators of dizziness and migraine episodes. When you go too long without eating, your blood sugar drops (a state called hypoglycemia), forcing your body to release stress hormones to compensate. This can worsen the sense of disequilibrium, lightheadedness, and increase vulnerability to migraine triggers.

Conversely, eating large, heavy meals, especially those high in sugar or refined carbohydrates, can cause a subsequent dip in blood sugar as the body produces excess insulin in response. These peaks and troughs create an unstable internal environment, which may sensitize the brain's migraine centers and destabilize the vestibular system.

Research demonstrates that individuals with migraine benefit from regular, balanced meals spaced throughout the day. This practice helps to maintain steady glucose levels, which supports both neurological health and the smooth functioning of balance pathways. The key message is to avoid skipping meals and prevent yourself from getting ravenously hungry.

Spacing Meals and Snacks to Maintain Vestibular Stability

The timing and spacing of your meals and snacks can directly influence how well your body manages energy, fluids, and neurological signaling. Experts suggest aiming for three balanced meals and two snacks per day, with no more than 3 to 4 hours between eating sessions. This frequent, predictable pattern reduces the chance of sudden glucose lows and helps keep electrolyte and fluid intake on track.

Here is a simple schedule you can try as a foundation:

- ***7:00 am***: Breakfast with water or herbal tea
- ***10:00 am***: Snack (nuts, yogurt, or fruit)
- ***12:30 pm***: Lunch with water
- ***3:00 pm***: Snack (vegetables with hummus, a boiled egg, or a small smoothie)
- ***6:30 pm***: Dinner with water
- ***Optional***: A light bedtime snack if 3 or more hours elapse between dinner and sleep.

Snacks should combine a source of protein, fiber, and some healthy fat to slow absorption and minimize glucose spikes. Examples include a handful of almonds with a piece of fruit, a rice cake with nut butter, or cooked chickpeas tossed with olive oil and herbs.

Keeping your meals and snacks on a schedule provides your vestibular system and brain with a steady fuel supply, minimizing one of the most controllable sources of dizziness and migraine flare-ups.

Tools for Tracking Fluid and Food Intake

Establishing these routines is the first step, but turning them into lasting habits requires awareness and tracking. Recording what and when you eat and drink, as well as noting symptoms, is a proven method for building insight and accountability. For beginners, many find it helpful to keep a dedicated hydration and meal log for at least 2 to 4 weeks as they experiment with hydration schedules and meal timing.

Tracking can be as simple or as advanced as you like:

- ***Pen and paper***: Maintain a notebook where you jot down the time and type of each drink or meal, along with a quick note about mood, symptoms, or notable events.

- ***Printable templates***: Use checklists or trackers found online; some headache and migraine support websites offer free resources you can print and keep handy.
- ***Mobile apps***: There are a variety of apps designed for tracking nutrition, fluid intake, and migraine symptoms. Look for those that let you set reminders, summarize data, and export reports to share with your healthcare provider.
- ***Integrated health logs***: If you already use a symptom tracking or health journal for your vestibular migraine triggers, simply add columns dedicated to tracking hydration, meal times, and snacks.

Tracking provides a double benefit because it supports habit formation and quickly reveals patterns. You may notice, for example, that on high-activity days or during warm weather, you are more prone to dizziness in the afternoons if you miss a snack or forget to hydrate between meals.

It can also help identify which electrolyte sources you tolerate best, and whether certain foods or eating schedules seem to lessen or aggravate your vestibular symptoms.

The simple acts of drinking enough fluids, incorporating natural electrolytes, and spreading meals and snacks consistently throughout the day form the core foundation for vestibular migraine stability. These habits strengthen your body's ability to maintain blood pressure, brain perfusion, and steady neurological function, all of which are critical for minimizing dizziness, vertigo, and other disruptive symptoms.

Creating a personalized hydration schedule, focusing on wholesome electrolyte sources, structuring regular meals and snacks, and tracking your progress will help you experience more consistent days and fewer unwelcome surprises. The next chapters will build on this solid foundation and introduce additional nutrition strategies and lifestyle adjustments for comprehensive migraine management.

Step 3 - Introducing Vestibular-Friendly Nutrition

After establishing stable hydration, balanced electrolytes, and a reliable meal schedule, the next step in managing vestibular migraine is to actively build a nutrient-dense, migraine-safe diet tailored for brain and vestibular system health. This chapter will walk you through the foods and nutrients with the best evidence for supporting neurological stability, explain how to foster a gut environment that helps reduce inflammation, and offer practical templates for meal planning and prep. You will learn how to confidently add foods that support symptom reduction, shifting the focus from simply avoiding triggers to embracing supportive nutrition.

Adding Migraine-Safe Nutrient-Dense Foods to Your Routine

Once common triggers like caffeine, aged cheeses, and processed meats have been reduced or eliminated, it is important to fill those gaps with foods that provide steady energy and promote healing. For individuals with vestibular migraine, "nutrient-dense" does not just mean foods packed with vitamins and minerals, but also those that avoid triggering the nervous system or inflaming the inner ear.

<u>Common migraine-safe, nutrient-rich foods include:</u>

- ***Leafy green vegetables***: Spinach, kale, and arugula.
- ***Non-citrus fruits***: Blueberries, pears, and apples.
- ***Root vegetables***: Sweet potatoes, carrots, and beets.
- ***Lean proteins***: Chicken, turkey, beans, and lentils.
- ***Whole gluten-free grains***: Quinoa, brown rice, and oats.
- ***Seeds and nuts***: Pumpkin seeds, chia seeds, and walnuts, as tolerated, since these can be triggers for some individuals.
- ***Healthy fats***: Extra-virgin olive oil and avocados.
- ***Fermented foods***: Plain yogurt, kefir, and sauerkraut, if tolerated.

Each person will have different levels of tolerance, so it is wise to reintroduce nutrient-dense foods in small amounts and keep tracking symptoms. The aim is to support your nervous system with consistent nutrition that minimizes the risk of sudden blood sugar drops, migraines, and dizziness flares.

Instead of focusing on restriction, try shifting your mindset to abundance. Adding a cup of spinach to your lunch, swapping white rice for quinoa, or using olive oil as your main cooking fat are small changes that can deliver significant nutritional payoffs over time.

Role of Magnesium, Riboflavin, and CoQ10 in Symptom Relief

Decades of research in migraine prevention point to three nutrients with particular promise: magnesium, riboflavin (vitamin B2), and coenzyme Q10 (CoQ10). All three play critical roles in energy production, nerve signaling, and protecting brain cells from oxidative stress. These factors are increasingly understood to be at the root of migraine mechanisms, including those affecting the vestibular pathways.

Magnesium is involved in over 300 biochemical reactions in the body, including nerve impulse transmission and blood vessel regulation. For migraines, magnesium may help calm overactive brain regions and reduce excitability that can lead to symptoms like dizziness and light sensitivity. Foods rich in magnesium include pumpkin seeds, Swiss chard, spinach, black beans, and cashews. Many people fall short of their daily magnesium needs, making dietary emphasis essential.

Riboflavin (Vitamin B2) supports mitochondrial function, the process your cells use to generate energy. Poor energy metabolism is a proposed factor in migraine susceptibility. Eating more riboflavin-rich foods like eggs, lean meats, fortified gluten-free cereals, and certain green vegetables can help meet your needs safely.

CoQ10 is a powerful antioxidant involved in mitochondrial health and has shown promising results in research on migraine frequency and severity. It is found in organ meats like liver and kidney, as well as in fatty fish, spinach, and whole grains. While supplements are available, dietary sources are a gentle way to support your nutrient status while tracking your body's response.

Nutrient Integration Guide

When trying to boost these nutrients through food, aim for the following daily targets:

- ***Magnesium***: At least two servings of magnesium-rich foods.
- ***Riboflavin***: At least one significant riboflavin source.
- ***CoQ10***: At least one CoQ10 source.

If you have dietary restrictions, such as veganism or food allergies, consider discussing supplementation with a healthcare professional.

Low-Glycemic Carbohydrates and Healthy Fats for Brain Health

Food choices that keep blood sugar stable are critical for anyone with vestibular migraine because sharp peaks and crashes in energy can trigger attacks. A low-glycemic diet emphasizes carbohydrates that break down slowly. This provides steady fuel to both your brain and the delicate inner ear structures.

Examples of low-glycemic carbs include:

- ***Legumes***: lentils, chickpeas, and black beans.
- ***Starchy vegetables***: sweet potato and squash.
- ***Grains***: quinoa, brown rice, and old-fashioned oats.
- ***Non-starchy vegetables***: green peas and other green greens.

Try to combine carbohydrates with a lean protein and healthy fat at every meal. This balance blunts the post-meal rise in blood sugar and helps you feel fuller longer. It also reduces the urge to snack on processed or sugary foods that may destabilize your nervous system.

The Importance of Healthy Fats

Healthy fats are more than just calorie dense. They are essential for building myelin, which is the protective sheath around nerves. They also help reduce inflammation and assist in absorbing fat-soluble vitamins needed for nervous system repair.

Focus especially on:

- ***Extra-virgin olive oil***
- ***Avocados***
- ***Nuts and seeds***: especially walnuts and chia seeds.

- ***Fatty fish***: such as salmon, sardines, or mackerel (if tolerated).

Intentionally including one serving of healthy fat at lunch and dinner (for example, a tablespoon of olive oil, half an avocado, or a handful of nuts) is an easy way to keep your brain fueled and your vestibular system steady throughout the day.

Gut-Brain Axis Considerations for Inflammation Reduction

Emerging research reveals that gut health and brain function are tightly intertwined, a relationship known as the gut-brain axis. The state of your gut microbiome can influence not only inflammation throughout the body but also the function and reactivity of the nervous system. This is especially relevant in vestibular migraine, where systemic inflammation and altered signaling between the gut and brain may exacerbate attacks.

Key gut-friendly practices that can support vestibular migraine management:

- ***Incorporating fermented foods***: such as plain yogurt, kefir, kimchi, or naturally fermented pickles, provided these do not trigger your symptoms.
- ***Increasing fiber***: through vegetables, fruits, whole gluten-free grains, and seeds. These feed beneficial gut

bacteria and promote the production of anti-inflammatory compounds.

- ***Favoring whole, unprocessed foods***: to limit artificial additives and preservatives which may disrupt the microbiome.
- ***Supporting prebiotics***: drinking adequate water and including prebiotic-rich foods like asparagus, onions, and leeks.

Some people with migraine have developed food sensitivities due to altered gut permeability. Pay attention to your symptoms and consider introducing new gut-friendly foods gradually. If you have a history of irritable bowel syndrome or significant digestive discomfort, individualized adjustments or consultation with a dietitian can be helpful.

Menu Templates and Meal Prep Strategies

Translating these guidelines into everyday meals is where many beginners get stuck. Consistency is key, and meal prep can make following a vestibular-friendly plan much more manageable. Start simple by batch preparing a few staple foods, like a quinoa salad, roasted sweet potatoes, or a pot of lentils. This gives you ready-made building blocks for meals throughout the week.

Here is a sample template for structuring vestibular-safe, nutrient-dense meals:

Breakfast Options:

- Oatmeal made with unsweetened almond milk, topped with blueberries, chia seeds, and a sprinkle of pumpkin seeds.
- Scrambled eggs with spinach and sautéed sweet potatoes.
- Plain Greek yogurt with sliced pears and a handful of walnuts.

Lunch Options:

- Quinoa salad with grilled chicken, kale, and pumpkin seeds, drizzled with olive oil and lemon juice (omit lemon if citrus sensitive).
- Brown rice bowl with black beans, roasted carrots, and avocado.
- Mixed leaf lettuce with tuna packed in olive oil, sliced apples, and sunflower seeds.

Dinner Options:

- Baked salmon or white fish with steamed broccoli, brown rice, and a drizzle of flaxseed oil.
- Lentil stew with carrots, celery, sweet potato, and arugula.
- Stir-fried tofu with snap peas, bok choy, brown rice noodles, and sesame oil.

Snack Ideas:

- A small handful of unsalted cashews and an apple.
- Hummus with carrot sticks and cucumber slices.
- Plain kefir, if dairy is tolerated, with chia seeds.

Effective Meal Prep Strategies

Meal prepping can be as simple as doubling recipes for lunch leftovers, washing and portioning veggies for quick snacks, or setting aside an hour each week to chop, roast, or cook basic ingredients. Use airtight containers to keep produce fresh and label meals for easy organization.

For grocery shopping, write your week's menu and list ingredients by store section. This keeps you focused on whole foods, prevents impulse buys of processed trigger foods, and saves time in the store. Stock your pantry with core "safe" foods such as gluten-free oats, brown rice, dried beans, and olive oil so you are always prepared to make a nourishing meal.

Finally, track how your body responds as you introduce these new foods and patterns. A food and symptom journal becomes especially informative as your diet expands to include more medicinal nutrients. With each week of practice, your confidence and consistency in making vestibular-friendly choices will grow.

Step 4 - Movement, Sleep Optimization, and Stress Management

Establishing a therapeutic lifestyle is a crucial piece in achieving consistent relief from vestibular migraine. After setting a foundation with dietary changes and steady hydration, it is time to turn your focus to everyday routines that impact your body and mind.

Three pillars, which are movement, sleep, and stress regulation, not only help reduce the frequency and severity of vestibular migraine symptoms but also build long-term resilience in your vestibular and nervous systems. Each element is approachable, even for total beginners. They can be seamlessly integrated into your daily life when you understand the basic principles and know where to start.

Vestibular Rehabilitation Exercises for Dizziness Reduction

For many people with vestibular migraine, dizziness, vertigo, and imbalance are among the most disabling symptoms.

Fortunately, the brain and vestibular system possess strong adaptive capabilities. Vestibular rehabilitation therapy (VRT) uses precise, gentle exercises to help retrain your brain to process movement and balance signals more accurately. This process, known as neuroplasticity, allows you to become less sensitive to triggers that would previously cause dizzy spells or unsteadiness.

Vestibular rehabilitation exercises come in different forms. The most common categories include:

1. **Gaze stabilization:**

   This often involves keeping your eyes fixed on a target while gently moving your head from side to side. For example, you might sit in a chair and, focusing on a sticker on the wall at eye level, slowly rotate your head right and left for 30 seconds at a time. This helps the brain communicate efficiently with the eye muscles and adapt to changes in head positioning.

2. **Balance training:**

   Exercises such as standing with feet together and eyes closed or gently shifting your weight from one foot to the other can gradually improve your sense of equilibrium.

3. **Habituation exercises:**

   These expose you, very slowly and carefully, to controlled versions of movements that typically provoke symptoms. With repeated practice, these exercises reduce your nervous system's overreaction to motion.

It is important that you start slowly, ideally under the supervision of a vestibular physiotherapist or using validated online resources, to avoid overloading your system and aggravating symptoms. Consistency is key. Practicing for five to ten minutes, two to three times daily, is often enough to make a noticeable difference over weeks.

Structuring a Gentle Exercise Routine for Vestibular Resilience

One challenge for people with vestibular migraine is that vigorous or erratic exercise may temporarily worsen dizziness or trigger symptoms. However, the right type of movement is an essential ingredient for long-term success. Gentle, regular exercise supports vestibular rehabilitation, enhances circulation to the brain, and buffers against the negative effects of chronic stress.

The best beginner routines focus on low-impact, steady activities that do not provoke symptoms. Walking, stationary cycling, gentle yoga, tai chi, and water aerobics are all effective starts. For instance, a daily 20-minute walk at a comfortable pace provides the dual benefit of movement and a stable visual environment. Yoga and tai chi improve balance, spatial awareness, and core strength. These are all factors that enhance your ability to navigate daily life with less fear of dizziness or falls.

Consider the following template for building your own vestibular-friendly fitness routine:

- ***Frequency***: Aim for two to five sessions per week, each lasting 15 to 30 minutes.
- ***Intensity***: Start with low-impact activities, increasing duration or intensity only when you feel secure.
- ***Balance Practice***: Incorporate simple balance drills, like standing on one leg near a support or practicing slow heel-to-toe walking.
- ***Adaptation***: If symptoms emerge, rest before trying again; gradual progression is both safe and effective.

Don't neglect the importance of warm-ups and cool-downs, and avoid sudden changes in direction or high-energy bursting activities until your system adapts. Keeping a brief exercise log can help you track both physical progress and any changes in vestibular symptoms.

Sleep Hygiene Techniques Tailored for Migraine Sensitivity

Sleep and vestibular migraine are tightly connected. Both sleep deprivation and irregular sleep patterns can lower your threshold for an attack, increase dizziness, and heighten sensitivity to environmental triggers. On the flip side, consistent and restorative sleep strengthens the brain's resilience, stabilizes mood, and reduces overall symptom burden.

For people struggling with vestibular migraine, a traditional approach to sleep hygiene needs specific tailoring. The following strategies can be effective:

- ***Strict sleep and wake schedules***: Go to bed and wake up at the same time every day, even on weekends. This consistency supports your circadian rhythms and lowers migraine risk.
- ***Prepare an optimal sleep environment***: Keep your room cool, dark, and quiet. Use blackout curtains or a sleep mask, and consider a white noise machine to reduce auditory disturbances.
- ***Screen-time management***: Avoid bright screens at least one hour before bedtime. Blue light can disrupt melatonin production, making it harder to both fall and stay asleep.
- ***Wind-down rituals***: Try reading, gentle stretches, or relaxation breathing before bed.

- ***Avoid food triggers and large meals close to bedtime***: Caffeine, chocolate, aged cheeses, or MSG, even in small quantities, may worsen nocturnal symptoms or provoke a rough morning.

For those who struggle to fall asleep because of vertigo or background dizziness, elevating your head slightly and using extra pillows for added neck support can sometimes reduce vestibular sensitivity in bed. Tracking your sleep and noting correlations with symptom flare-ups can provide essential clues for further refinement.

Stress Modulation Strategies Specific to Vestibular Symptoms

Stress is a well-documented precipitating factor for both migraine and vestibular dysfunction. The body's fight-or-flight response can amplify neurotransmitter imbalances, heighten sensitivity to environmental changes, and increase muscle tension in the neck and shoulders. All of these factors can fuel vestibular migraine attacks or prolong recovery times.

Stress management must be practical and feasible. Techniques that specifically help people with vestibular migraine include:

- ***Identifying stressors***: Use a symptom diary to track what events, environments, or emotions are most often linked to dizziness flare-ups.

- ***Planning rest breaks***: Build short, frequent rest periods into your day, particularly before or after challenging activities. Even five minutes of quiet time can help reset a hyper-aroused nervous system.
- ***Progressive muscle relaxation***: This involves systematically tensing and relaxing muscle groups, focusing especially on neck, shoulders, and jaw muscles.
- ***Breathing exercises***: Slow, abdominal breathing can reduce the body's overall stress response and stabilize heart rate and blood pressure. Try a simple four-count inhale and six-count exhale pattern for three minutes at a time.
- ***Support networks***: Engage with migraine-focused support groups in person or online. Social connection can provide encouragement and practical tips, reducing the mental burden of chronic symptoms.

If you notice specific stressors are consistently tied with increases in dizziness or headache severity, consider discussing these patterns with your healthcare provider or a counselor who understands migraine disorders. Cognitive behavioral strategies, like reframing anxious thoughts about symptom triggers, may be especially effective for building long-term coping capacity.

Integrating Mindfulness and Relaxation Practices

Mindfulness-based practices have gained attention as valuable adjuncts in migraine and vestibular care. Such practices help quiet the nervous system, reduce hypervigilance, and break the cycle of worry that often accompanies unpredictable symptoms. The foundational principle is to develop greater awareness and acceptance of both physical and emotional experiences, allowing the body to shift from a reactive to a regulated state.

Here are ways to incorporate mindfulness and relaxation into your routine:

- ***Start with brief body scans***: Set aside five minutes to mentally scan and acknowledge sensations throughout your body without judgment, beginning at your toes and moving to your head.
- ***Guided meditation***: Use audio recordings or meditation apps designed for beginners. Techniques might include focusing on your breath, repeating calming phrases, or visualizing serene, stable environments.
- ***Grounding exercises***: When dizziness strikes, focus on the sensations of your feet against the floor or tightly grip a comforting object. This can anchor your attention in the present moment and reduce anxiety-driven escalation.

- ***Gentle yoga and mindful movement***: These combine physical stability with mental focus, doubling as both exercise and relaxation practice.

It is not necessary to meditate for long periods; even two to five minutes twice daily can provide cumulative benefits and build a sense of control over your internal state. Many people find that pairing mindfulness with other lifestyle modifications, such as improved sleep and gentle exercise, amplifies overall resilience.

In putting these strategies together, remember that progress is gradual. Small, consistent changes often yield powerful long-term improvements in how your body handles dizziness, fatigue, and stress. Pay attention to what works for you and give yourself credit for each positive step.

Step 5 - Targeted Supplements and Herbal Approaches

For many living with vestibular migraine, navigating through diet, exercise, and stress management creates a strong foundation for natural management. However, nutrition alone may not provide complete symptom relief, and some individuals benefit from the addition of supplements or herbal supports.

This chapter guides you through the evidence-based use of targeted supplements and selected herbal approaches as part of a comprehensive vestibular migraine action plan. You'll learn which options have robust research support, how to select high-quality products, and crucial steps to take before introducing new supplements into your regimen.

Herbal Options: Butterbur, Feverfew, Ginger, and Their Safety Profiles

In addition to vitamins and minerals, a variety of herbal remedies have been researched for their potential to support individuals with migraine, including vestibular migraine.

Among the herbal options, butterbur (Petasites hybridus), feverfew (Tanacetum parthenium), and ginger are most frequently discussed due to their promising effects and accessibility. Each herb has a distinct profile in terms of efficacy, usage, and safety. This is important for those considering these supplements as part of their migraine management plan.

Below is a detailed discussion of these three herbal options, including their benefits, recommended forms, and crucial safety considerations:

1. **Butterbur (Petasites hybridus)**
    - ***Potential Benefits***: Research suggests that butterbur may help decrease the frequency and severity of migraine attacks. Some clinical trials have demonstrated that standardized butterbur extract, when taken regularly, can offer significant preventive benefits.
    - ***Safety Profile***: A critical safety note is that only butterbur products labeled as "PA-free" (pyrrolizidine alkaloid-free) should be considered. Pyrrolizidine alkaloids are naturally occurring toxins present in some butterbur preparations and are known to cause serious liver damage.
    - ***Dosage and Use***: PA-free butterbur supplements are typically available in capsule

form. While short-term use under medical supervision may be beneficial, the long-term safety of butterbur remains unclear.

- ***Precautions***: Individuals with liver disease or those taking medications that affect liver function should avoid butterbur. Consultation with a healthcare provider is essential.

2. **Feverfew (Tanacetum parthenium)**
   - ***Potential Benefits***: Feverfew has a long history of traditional use for headache relief. Some modern studies support its role in reducing migraine frequency and severity, though research results are mixed.
   - ***Safety Profile***: Feverfew is generally considered safe for short-term use, but it may cause gastrointestinal side effects such as nausea, bloating, or mouth ulcers.
   - ***Special Considerations***: Feverfew should be avoided during pregnancy due to its potential to stimulate uterine contractions. It can also increase bleeding risk, especially when combined with blood-thinning medications like warfarin or aspirin.
   - ***Dosage and Use***: Feverfew is available in capsule, tablet, or tea form. Consistency in dosing and product quality is important.

3. **Ginger (Zingiber officinale)**
   - ***Potential Benefits***: Ginger is well-known for its anti-nausea properties and mild anti-inflammatory effects. Studies have shown that ginger can be effective in relieving acute migraine attacks and managing vestibular symptoms, such as nausea and dizziness.
   - ***Safety Profile***: Ginger is generally safe when used in culinary amounts. In supplement form, it is well-tolerated by most, but high doses may increase bleeding risk.
   - ***Dosage and Use***: Ginger can be consumed fresh, as a powder, in capsules, or as tea. It offers a convenient, natural option for symptom relief during acute episodes.

Table: Summary Table of Herbal Supplement Considerations

Herb	**Primary Use**	**Key Safety Note**
Butterbur	Prevention	***Must be PA-free*** to avoid liver toxicity.
Feverfew	Prevention	Avoid in pregnancy and with blood thinners.
Ginger	Nausea/Acute Relief	Generally safe; use caution with bleeding disorders.

General Guidelines for Herbal Supplement Use

- Always select products from reputable sources that provide clear purity statements and adhere to manufacturing standards.

- Discuss any herbal supplement use with a healthcare provider, especially if you have underlying health conditions or take prescription medications.
- Monitor for potential side effects and discontinue use if adverse reactions occur.

Professional guidance is strongly recommended when incorporating these herbs into your migraine management plan.

Evaluating Supplement Quality and Avoiding Interactions

Quality assurance is one of your strongest defenses against ineffective or harmful supplements. Always research supplement brands for third-party testing, customer reviews, and recall history.

Look for seals from ***USP*** (United States Pharmacopeia), ***NSF International***, or ***ConsumerLab***. These logos indicate that a product has been independently tested for its contents and purity.

- ***Check Inactive Ingredients***: Review the label and watch for additives that may themselves be migraine triggers. These include artificial dyes or preservatives.
- ***The "Natural" Myth***: Be aware that “natural” does not always mean safe or effective. In the world of supplements, more is not necessarily better.

Managing Interactions and Risks

It is essential to recognize that supplements can interact with one another and with prescription medications. For example, some herbal supplements can affect blood clotting or liver function. Others may impact the absorption or effectiveness of antibiotics, antidepressants, or seizure medications.

Always keep a detailed record of all supplements and medications you are taking, and update it whenever you make a change.

Special Medical Considerations

If you have underlying health conditions, such as kidney disease, liver disease, or cardiovascular disorders, careful medical oversight is particularly important. Supplements may worsen these conditions or interact with drugs prescribed for their management.

Because regulations for dietary supplements are less strict than for medications, it is wise to err on the side of caution. Adopt a ***"start low, go slow"*** approach when introducing anything new to your routine.

Consultation Protocols Before Starting Supplementation

Before adding any supplement or herbal remedy to your regimen, especially if you currently take prescription drugs or have chronic health conditions, it is important to consult a healthcare professional. The best practice is to discuss your full health history, current symptoms, medication list, and your interest in supplements with either your primary care physician, a neurologist experienced in vestibular migraine, or a registered dietitian specializing in migraine care.

Bring labels, ingredient lists, and dosing plans to your consultation for a thorough review. Ask about potential benefits, side effects, and risks of interactions with your current medications. If your care provider is unfamiliar with a supplement, request a referral to someone with integrative or functional medicine experience, or a pharmacist who has expertise in supplement-drug interactions.

Setting Goals and Expectations

During your consultation, clarify your goals. Are you seeking fewer vestibular migraine attacks, less severe symptoms, or better control of dizziness and fatigue?

- ***Set Trial Timelines***: Most migraine supplements may require 2 to 3 months before full effects are seen.
- ***Establish Check-ins***: Schedule regular follow-ups to assess progress and adapt your approach as needed.
- ***Safety First***: Document any new or worsening symptoms after starting a supplement, and suspend use if adverse reactions appear.

A collaborative approach ensures that your supplement choices are safe, evidence-based, and tailored to your unique vestibular needs.

Practical Steps to Get Started

To put this guidance into practice, consider the following approach:

1. Identify your primary goals (for example: reducing migraine days, controlling daily dizziness, or addressing fatigue).
2. Research and shortlist the supplement(s) or herbal remedy most likely to benefit your specific symptom profile.
3. Look for pharmaceutical or third-party certified brands, checking for the most bioavailable forms and appropriate dosages.
4. Consult with your healthcare provider for a thorough risk-benefit assessment and interaction review.
5. Track your symptoms and supplement intake using a dedicated journal for at least eight to twelve weeks.
6. Regularly assess with your provider and adjust or discontinue as needed based on your body's response.

Remember that supplements and herbs are most effective when incorporated as part of a broader plan, working in combination with dietary modifications, hydration, adequate sleep, gentle movement, and stress reduction. They are not substitutes for these foundations; instead, they serve as targeted aids to amplify your recovery and support long-term relief from vestibular migraine.

Crafting Your Sustainable Vestibular Migraine Action Plan

Bringing together dietary changes, lifestyle adjustments, and targeted supplements forms a powerful toolkit for managing vestibular migraine. But understanding each of these pieces isn't enough on its own. Lasting improvement relies on weaving them into a realistic, personalized plan that supports you day by day, adapts to your progress, and connects you to sources of support and reliable information.

This chapter will guide you through the process of synthesizing the information from previous chapters into an actionable, sustainable vestibular migraine action plan tailored to your needs.

Synthesizing dietary, lifestyle, and supplement strategies

Effective management of vestibular migraine means addressing multiple aspects of your daily routine. Diet is a central pillar: consistently avoiding known triggers, supporting hydration and electrolyte balance, prioritizing vestibular-friendly foods, and ensuring you receive key nutrients are all essential steps.

Beyond what you eat, your lifestyle, which includes how you move, sleep, and manage stress, plays a crucial role. Regular, gentle exercise and vestibular rehabilitation exercises help maintain balance and reduce dizziness episodes. Sleep hygiene and stress reduction, such as mindfulness or breathing practices, support stability in your nervous system. Supplements can complement this foundation by targeting common deficiencies associated with migraine and vestibular symptoms. Research highlights the benefits of magnesium, riboflavin (vitamin B2), and CoQ10 in reducing migraine frequency and severity. Herbal options such as ginger or feverfew may provide additional support when chosen carefully and in consultation with your healthcare provider.

The key is not to treat each strategy in isolation, but to integrate them so each component reinforces the others. When your diet, habits, and supplements align, your body's threshold for migraine symptoms may improve. This allows you to gain a greater sense of agency over your condition.

Creating a Personalized Plan with SMART Health Goals

A generic plan is rarely effective for complex, variable conditions like vestibular migraine. Tailoring your approach begins with setting clear, measurable objectives using the

SMART framework: Specific, Measurable, Achievable, Relevant, and Time-bound.

Here is how you can develop your personal vestibular migraine action plan:

1. **Reflect on your priorities:**

   Which symptoms bother you most? Do you want more energy, fewer dizzy spells, or better concentration?

2. **Review your data:**

   Look over your symptom and food diary. Note patterns, triggers, and any helpful interventions identified so far.

3. **Set 2 to 3 initial SMART goals:**
   - ***Specific***: "I will eliminate caffeine and aged cheese for the next four weeks and monitor any changes in dizziness using my diary."
   - ***Measurable***: "I will add a daily 10-minute vestibular exercise routine, five days per week, tracked on my calendar."
   - ***Time-bound***: "Starting this week, I will take a pharmaceutical-grade magnesium supplement (as guided by my doctor) every day for the next two months."

4. **Break larger goals into manageable steps:**

   If stress is a major trigger, your first step might be scheduling a 5-minute relaxation practice at midday. This is more effective than trying to overhaul your entire routine overnight.

5. **Set review dates:**

   Mark your calendar at two and four week milestones. Use these times to check in on your progress and make adjustments as needed.

Personalizing your plan keeps you motivated and focused. It allows you to measure your success with each specific, achievable goal. Using this deliberate approach transforms wishful thinking into actionable progress.

Monitoring and Adapting to Symptom Changes Over Time

Vestibular migraine symptoms can change in intensity and character over weeks or months. Factors like life circumstances, stress, hormonal cycles, and even weather patterns can influence these shifts. Maintaining a consistent tracking system is crucial to adapt your action plan accordingly.

Here are practical tools for staying in tune with your progress:

- ***Continue your logs***: Use a symptom and food diary or a digital tracking app to record meals, exercise, sleep, supplement intake, and daily symptoms.
- ***Identify patterns***: Note patterns of improvement or flare-ups. Try to link them to recent changes in diet, routine, or external stressors.
- ***Analyze setbacks***: If you experience setbacks, review your logs for missed triggers, inconsistent hydration, or lapses in sleep routine. Remember that one-off episodes are common even with good adherence. However, frequent setbacks may signal the need to re-examine your plan with a professional.
- ***Practice self-compassion***: Be honest and gentle with yourself during this process. View adjustments as a natural part of managing a chronic health condition rather than failures.

If a particular food or lifestyle change leads to improvement, make it a permanent part of your plan. If something does not yield a benefit after a fair trial (typically 4 to 8 weeks for dietary and supplement changes), reconsider its place in your regimen.

Building Social and Clinical Support Networks

Successful long-term management of vestibular migraine is rarely a solo endeavor. Building a network of social, clinical, and informational support can help you stay accountable, motivated, and resilient.

Start by considering the following support resources:

- ***Family and Friends***: Educate your loved ones about vestibular migraine and your action plan. Ask for their help with meal planning, maintaining a calm environment, or simply providing understanding on difficult days.
- ***Healthcare Providers***: Maintain regular check-ins with your primary care doctor, headache specialist, or neurologist. Share your symptom logs and progress updates to help guide safe medication adjustments or therapy referrals.
- ***Vestibular Therapists***: If balance or dizziness remains a primary symptom, seek a referral to a vestibular rehabilitation specialist. These professionals provide tailored exercises and progress monitoring to reduce vestibular symptoms.
- ***Peer Support Groups***: Online and in-person communities, such as those provided by vestibular advocacy organizations, can offer invaluable encouragement and problem-solving. Sharing experiences reduces isolation and can spark new ideas for managing triggers.
- ***Migraine Associations***: Organizations like the Vestibular Disorders Association (VeDA) and the American Migraine Foundation offer webinars, articles, and directories of specialists to help you stay abreast of new research.

Remember that your support network is not static. Let it expand or change as your needs evolve. Asking for help, scheduling regular check-ins, or participating in support forums can make challenging periods far more manageable.

Resources for Continued Learning and Accountability

Vestibular migraine research and best practices continue to evolve. Staying informed will empower you to adapt your action plan as the landscape changes, ensuring access to emerging treatments or strategies.

Explore the following resources for ongoing education and self-advocacy:

- ***The American Migraine Foundation***: This organization maintains an extensive library of patient guides, dietary resources, and research news curated for non-clinicians.
- ***The Vestibular Disorders Association (VeDA)***: This is a premier resource that offers condition-specific articles, symptom trackers, video tutorials for vestibular exercises, and directories of support groups.
- ***The National Institutes of Health (NIH) MedlinePlus***: This site provides accessible explanations and updates on migraine, vestibular disorders, and related treatments.
- ***Migraine Tracking Apps***: Tools such as Migraine Buddy or N-1 Headache help you document symptoms

and trigger exposures over time. These apps generate progress reports for personal review or provider appointments.

- ***Your Care Team***: Regularly consult your doctors about new treatments, supplements, or exercise modalities. New research into non-pharmaceutical therapies, such as neuromodulation devices and expanded dietary protocols, is ongoing.

Accountability is just as important as education. Consider sharing your progress and goals with a trusted friend, family member, or support group to stay on track. Many people find value in periodic “self-audits.” These are brief monthly check-ins used to celebrate gains and troubleshoot challenges. Staying connected to both the latest research and your personal support system, you create a sustainable path toward long-term relief and stability.

Managing vestibular migraine is a dynamic process, not a one-time event. By integrating dietary, lifestyle, and supplement strategies, setting SMART health goals, monitoring your progress, and seeking social and clinical support, you establish a strong foundation for progress. Commit to ongoing learning, stay curious, and don’t hesitate to ask for help. Over time, the small daily actions you take will accumulate, leading to greater balance, confidence, and control over your health.

Conclusion

As we conclude this guide, it is worth reflecting on the practical, stepwise plan outlined throughout the previous chapters. Beginning with foundational education about what vestibular migraine is and how it uniquely manifests, you moved through clear steps: learning to track your symptoms and triggers, adopting a migraine-friendly dietary strategy, focusing on proper hydration and meal timing, enriching your diet with vestibular-supportive nutrients, implementing gentle movement and stress reduction techniques, and, when appropriate, incorporating targeted supplements for further support. Each of these steps builds on the last, designed to give you tools that address the underlying drivers of vestibular migraine instead of just the symptoms.

Following this plan offers numerous benefits. Identifying your personal triggers empowers you to make informed choices that reduce the occurrence of dizziness, vertigo, and migraine attacks. Adopting a consistent, balanced eating and hydration routine stabilizes your neurological system and minimizes surprise exacerbations. Practicing vestibular rehabilitation exercises and optimizing sleep hygiene gradually improve your baseline resilience.

The inclusion of evidence-based supplements offers extra support, particularly for persistent symptoms that diet and lifestyle alone may not fully address. Most importantly, this integrative approach encourages a sense of control and agency, replacing uncertainty with actionable knowledge.

However, it's important to understand that recovery from vestibular migraine rarely follows a linear path. Symptoms can wax and wane, and the effect of dietary or lifestyle changes may sometimes take several weeks or even months to become apparent. Adaptability is vital. What works for you during one period of life may need to be adjusted as your body, environment, or stress levels change. Frustration is natural, but patience plays a major role in long-term success. Setting realistic expectations and celebrating small victories help to sustain motivation through setbacks.

Being proactive in managing vestibular migraine is key to ongoing improvement. Regularly update your symptom and food diaries, review your action plan, and stay aware of new or recurring triggers. Keep your support network engaged, whether that includes friends, family, healthcare providers, or peer groups through advocacy organizations.. Don't hesitate to reach out for professional guidance when evaluating supplements, troubleshooting difficult symptoms, or when your needs change.

Ongoing education is another cornerstone of effective long-term management. The landscape of migraine care continues to evolve, with new research highlighting dietary connections, lifestyle modifications, and therapeutic options each year. Consult reputable organizations and specialist vestibular resources for updates, and empower yourself to ask informed questions at medical appointments. Every new insight you gain builds confidence and reinforces your capacity to make the best choices for your own health.

Controlling vestibular migraine is not always straightforward, but it is entirely possible. Following a structured, step-by-step plan, approaching recovery with adaptability and patience, and committing to proactive symptom management can help reduce your symptom burden and allow you to reclaim a greater quality of life. Every step forward, no matter how small, stands as a testament to your self-advocacy and resilience.

FAQs

How is vestibular migraine diagnosed?

Vestibular migraine is diagnosed primarily based on a detailed medical history and a careful assessment of symptoms. There is no single definitive test for vestibular migraine, so healthcare providers rely on diagnostic criteria established by organizations such as the International Headache Society and the Bárány Society.

Typically, diagnosis involves ruling out other causes of dizziness, such as inner ear disorders, and looking for a pattern of repeated episodes of vertigo or dizziness associated with migraine features (such as sensitivity to light, sound, or a history of migraines). Additional tests, like hearing exams, balance assessments, and brain imaging, may be ordered to exclude other conditions. Keeping a record of your symptoms can greatly assist your provider in making an accurate diagnosis.

Are there specific risk factors for developing vestibular migraine?

Certain risk factors can increase the likelihood of developing vestibular migraine. These include a personal or family history of migraine (with or without aura), being female, and experiencing hormonal fluctuations, such as those related to menstruation, pregnancy, or menopause. Stress, poor sleep, and certain lifestyle factors may also contribute. Genetics appear to play a significant role, as vestibular migraine tends to run in families. Understanding your risk factors can help you and your provider develop strategies to reduce your chances of experiencing frequent or severe episodes.

What lifestyle changes can help manage vestibular migraine?

Adopting healthy lifestyle habits is a cornerstone of vestibular migraine management. Regular sleep schedules, consistent meals, and stress-reducing activities such as yoga or meditation can decrease the frequency and severity of episodes. Avoiding known triggers, whether dietary, environmental, or emotional, can make a significant difference. Physical activity tailored to your tolerance (like walking or gentle stretching) may also help, as long as it doesn't provoke symptoms. Tracking these changes and their effects can provide valuable feedback for ongoing management.

Can vestibular migraine impact daily activities or work performance?

Yes, vestibular migraine can significantly interfere with daily life, including work, school, and social activities. Symptoms like dizziness, vertigo, and mental fogginess can make it difficult to concentrate, perform tasks, or participate in physical activities. Some individuals may need to adjust their work schedules, seek accommodations, or reduce exposure to environments that trigger symptoms (such as bright lights or loud noises). Communicating with employers, teachers, or family members about your condition can help you receive the support you need to manage your responsibilities effectively.

How does vestibular migraine affect mental health?

Living with vestibular migraine can have an emotional impact, sometimes leading to anxiety, depression, or feelings of isolation, especially if symptoms are frequent or severe. The unpredictability of episodes can create additional stress and worry. Support from mental health professionals, migraine support groups, and close communication with your healthcare provider can make a difference. Incorporating stress management strategies and seeking help when needed are important steps for maintaining emotional well-being.

Are children or adolescents affected by vestibular migraine?

Vestibular migraine is not limited to adults; children and adolescents can also be affected, although it may be underrecognized in younger individuals. In children, symptoms may present as episodes of dizziness, unexplained falls, or difficulty focusing in school, sometimes without the classic headache component. Pediatricians or pediatric neurologists can help assess and manage vestibular migraine in younger patients. Early recognition and intervention can improve outcomes and reduce the impact on school performance and daily life.

What is the long-term outlook for people with vestibular migraine?

The course of vestibular migraine varies from person to person. Some individuals experience periods of remission, while others may have persistent or recurring symptoms. With appropriate management, such as lifestyle adjustments, trigger avoidance, and, when necessary, medication, many people are able to significantly reduce the frequency and severity of episodes. Ongoing research continues to improve understanding and treatment of the condition, offering hope for better long-term outcomes. Regular follow-up with your healthcare provider is important to adapt your management plan as needed.

References and Helpful Links

Academic journal articles on vestibular migraine:. Retrieved January 23, 2026, from https://www.ncbi.nlm.nih.gov/pmc/articles/PMC3615450/

Migraine diet and nutrition research:. Retrieved January 23, 2026, from https://americanmigrainefoundation.org/resource-library/diet-and-headache/

Vestibular rehabilitation resources:. Retrieved January 23, 2026, from https://vestibular.org/resources/

Supplement efficacy studies:. Retrieved January 23, 2026, from https://www.ncbi.nlm.nih.gov/pmc/articles/PMC5871216/

Lempert, T. (n.d.). (n.d.). & Neuhauser, H.. Epidemiology of vertigo, migraine and vestibular migraine. Retrieved January 23, 2026, from https://scispace.com/pdf/epidemiology-of-vertigo-migraine-and-vestibular-migraine-4qcl9ogviw.pdf

Chiu, H. (n.d.). (n.d.). Y. et al.. Effect of magnesium on migraine: A systematic review. Retrieved January 23, 2026, from https://pubmed.ncbi.nlm.nih.gov/26752497/

Supplement efficacy studies: (n.d.). Supplement efficacy studies:. Retrieved January 23, 2026, from https://pmc.ncbi.nlm.nih.gov/articles/PMC8431076/

www.ingramcontent.com/pod-product-compliance
Lightning Source LLC
LaVergne TN
LVHW022015200926
848481LV00007B/2397